ALL ABOUT REIKI

By
Lena Sheehan

Earth Wise Books

ISBN-13:978-1539070498
ISBN-10:1539070492

First edition print published by Raular Publishing 2008
First edition eBook published by Black Horse Books
2012

 A note from the publisher

This Book is licensed for your personal enjoyment only
and is offered at a fair and reasonable cost. If you would
like to share this book with another person, please pur-
chase an additional copy for each reader. Thank you for
respecting the hard work of this author.

"Those who are drawn to Reiki and other types of healing modalities are those who listen to the whispers of the higher self - instead of the shouting and boasting of the ego."

Unknown

Contents

Lena Sheehan's Reiki Lineage

Reiki First and Second Degree
- Hawayo Takata
- Barbara Weber Ray
- Marsha Smith
- Barbara Roberts
- Eileen (Lena) Sheehan

Reiki Third Degree
- Hawayo Takata
- Ethel Lombardi
- Gail Fayhe
- Ed Michaud
- Barbara Roberts
- Eileen (Lena) Sheehan

Masters initiated by Grand Master Hawayo Takata

Although there may be more, the list be-low is the names of the 22 people who are known and recognized to have been initiated by Grand Master Hawayo Takata during her lifetime.

George Araki
Dorothy Baba
Ursula Baylow
Rick Bockner
Barbara Brown
Fran Brown
Patricia Ewing
Phyllis Lei Furumoto (Takata's granddaughter)

Beth Gray
John Gray
Iris Ishikura
Harry Kuboi
Ethel Lombardi
Mary McFadyen
Paul Mitchell
Bethel Phaigh
Barbara Weber Ray
Shinobu Saito
Virginia Samdahl
Wanja Twan
and Takata's Sister

Introduction

This book has been written for the purpose of providing all seekers of Reiki the Usui Shiki Ryoho method of Reiki as taught to me and as close to the original method as by Grand Master Hawayo Takata and handed down from generation to generation. It is in no way intended to replace actual instruction by a qualified Reiki Master Teacher.

As with many things in life, some students who learned this original method of Reiki felt they could expand and enhance what was and branched off to create their own version of Reiki. This explains why there are so many viewpoints on how Reiki should be performed and sanctified.

I can generally spot someone who was taught an "offshoot" from the original teachings simply by asking him or her lineage. If they are not able to quickly give it to me, it generally means they were taught one of the off branch versions of Reiki and not the actual version that was originally brought to the United States by Grand Master Takata. They also tend to not be aware of the respect that is traditionally paid to a Reiki Master from a level I or a level II practitioner; that teaching seems to have faded away. Another way is by the actually "feel" of the Reiki energy being channeled through the practitioner. Many have reported to me that it feels different to them when they have a Reiki session with a student from one of the Masters who is not of pure lineage. This does not mean that it is not effective, just that it feels different.

Grand Master Takata was of Japanese origin,

therefore she honored and respected the sacredness of the symbols, which were forbidden to be written down and required memorization. A student of direct lineage from Hawayo Takata, I held fast to the original teachings of no Reiki information should be put into print for many years. But, as time goes by and more and more books are popping up around the planet, my stubbornness and respect for the old ways seems futile.

So, in my desire to make certain the original method of Reiki that was taught to me to my students and all seekers, I have created this manual.

Having so stated, I want to also point out that you should go to whomever you are drawn to for your Reiki attunement and not necessarily to someone of direct lineage. Why? Because we are all individuals with a unique vibration and although the system may vary slightly from teacher to teacher all teachings of Reiki have validity. Whichever teacher you are drawn to is the perfect teacher for you. I encourage you to study and learn the original teachings but be true to your own vibrations for the actual attunement.

May you discover within these pages the magic and wonder that goes along with the phenomenon of Reiki.

First Degree Reiki

What is Reiki?

I can remember the very first time I was exposed to Reiki. I was working at a meta-physical function and chatting with the organizer when a man and woman across the room caught my eye. The woman was sitting peacefully in a chair while the man held his hands a few inches above her head. I watched with amazement as waves of energy flowed from his hands into the crown of her head. I immediately lost all train of thought for my conversation and stood speechless, watching. When I finally came to my senses and ask the organizer if she knew what the man was doing, she answered "Reiki". I knew right then that this was something I wanted to pursue.

Now, I will admit that most people are not able to see the energy as I did, but there are very few people indeed who can't feel it. Reiki is energy and energy always shows up in some tangible form. For me it was visual, for others it is feeling and yet others simply balance... but it is always felt.

The word Reiki (pronounced Rey - Key) is a Japanese word which means Universal Life Force Energy. This same meaning is Leiki (Lay -Key) in Chinese and the calligraphy (or Kanji) is the same for both the Japanese Reiki and the Chinese Leiki since both words originated in Tibet.

The top of the Japanese word, Rei, means: spirit or soul or ghost. The Chinese interpretation of Lei means: subtle influence; a force; ethereal or supernatural power. The original Tibetan source views it as the spirit of an entity that acts on others and is supernatural, efficacious and clever.

My Reiki Master told her class that she felt every human being on hearth does Reiki, but some just don't realize it. I agree. Just think for a minute. If you stub your toe or bang your head, what is the first thing you do? You place your hand over the wound and rub it or hold it there, correct? How about when someone you love gets injured? Don't you do the same for them? And doesn't this simple gesture of placing your hand over a wound somehow lessen the trauma and/or the pain? Everyone does it. It is a natural inherent instinct within every human being to utilize his or her own healing abilities.

Your hands can and do project energy. When you are injured and the desire to heal enters your thoughts, you pull to you the Universal Life Force Energy (Reiki) and it flows through your hands and into the wounded area. By being attuned to Reiki and learning the correct method of directing this energy you can help yourself or someone you love more effectively than the simple rub would do.

Kirlian photography refers to a form of contact print photography. It is named after Semyon Kirlian, who in 1939 accidentally discovered that if an object on a photographic plate is subjected to a strong electric field, an image is created on the plate Kirlian's work rediscovered a phenomenon and technique variously called "electrography," "electro photography," and "corona discharge photography."

The Kirlian Camera was used in the photos (pg. 11) to demonstrate the effects of Reiki. Photo number one is the prints of fingers prior to the activation of the Reiki energy. Photo number two is the print of the same fingers after the Reiki energy has been activated.

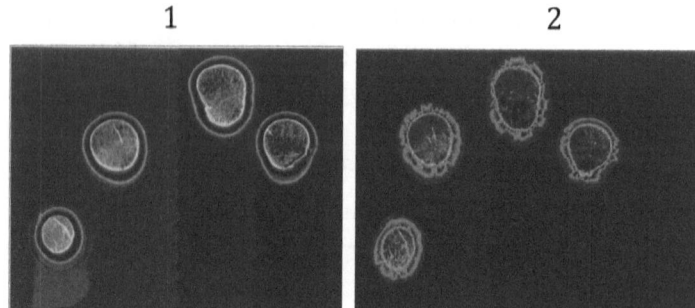

Before Reiki activation   After Reiki activation

Providing the masses with a photo of what Reiki looks like is much easier than explaining what it feels like.

Reiki is an ancient healing art form that taps into and directs the Universal Life Force Energy so that it can channel through the practitioner and bring forth balance and harmony. This allows the person, animal or plant (yes... plant!) to heal itself. A reiki practitioner is a healing facilitator, not a healer. As a facilitator, they allow the recipient to heal itself which it already knows how to do. Balance and harmony are our natural way of being and dis-ease comes from imbalances in our bodies. The really great thing about Reiki is that it has to go through the facilitator to reach the recipient. Because of this, the facilitator receives the benefits as well. This is truly a win-win situation!

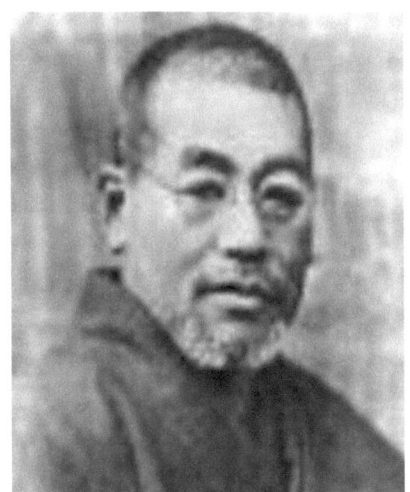

Dr. Mikao Usui
Re-discovered Reiki

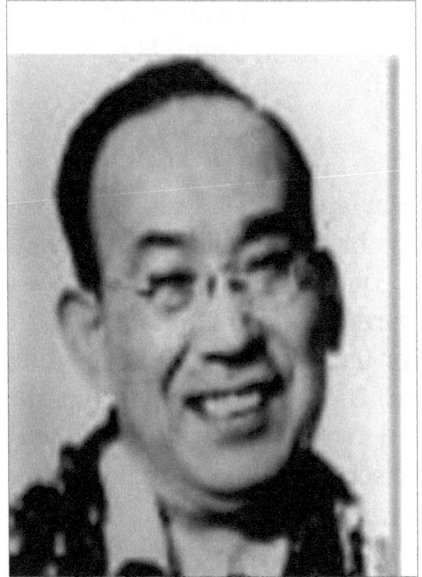

Dr.. Chujiro Hiyashi
Reiki Grand Master
1879-1941

Mrs. Hawayo Takata and Reiki

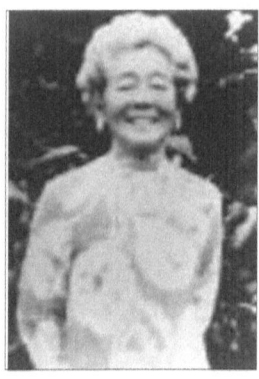

Mrs. Hawayo Takata
Reiki Grand Master
1900 - 1980

Mrs. Hawayo Takata was the Grand Master who is credited for bringing Reiki to the United States. She was born on December 24,1900 in Hawaii of Japanese immigrant parents and was named after the country of her birth. Her parents were pineapple cutters on the island of Kauai, Hawaii at Honolulu but Hawayo was too small and frail for plantation work so she took jobs while still in public school helping teach younger children and worked as a soda fountain clerk.

When she finished school, she was offered a servant's position at the large and wealthy plantation owner's house. She lived at the plantation for the next twenty-four years as a housekeeper and eventually a bookkeeper.

Hawayo met and married the plantation's accountant, Saichi Takata in 1917 and was quite happy. Saichi died in October, 1930 of a heart attack at the youthful age of 31 leaving Mrs. Takata was widowed with two small daughters. She worked hard to care for her children and soon became very ill. At the age of 35 years and weighing only 97 pounds, her small and delicate frame was burdened with appendicitis, a benign tumor, gallstones and asthma. She was unable to undergo any surgery which required anesthesia.

To add to her troubles, one of her family members died each year. Her parents had just returned to Japan for an extended visit of a year at their family home when her sister died. Mrs. Takata felt the news should be delivered to her parents in person so she took her children and went to Japan to tell them herself. There it was decided that she should try to regain her health by resting and eating well so that her body would be strong enough to undergo surgery. She went to visit a friend, Dr. T. Maeda, at the Maeda Orthopedic Hospital in the Akasaka district of Tokyo. Dr. Maeda invited Mrs. Takata, and her two daughters, to stay at the hospital while she healed.

After 21 days she was deemed strong enough to undergo the surgery she needed. It was scheduled and she was taken into the operating room and prepped for the surgery.

A voice rang loud and clear in Mrs. Takata's head, "Do not have the operation. It is not necessary." She got up off the table with the sheet wrapped around her. This caused quite a stir among the nurses as she asked Dr. Maeda if there was any other form of treatment she could have. He replied that there was, but it would depend on how long she could stay in Japan. He could not say whether the treatment would take two weeks, two months or a year. Mrs. Takata answered that she could stay for two years, so Dr. Maeda told her to get dressed and he called his sister, Mrs. Shimura, who was the hospital's dietitian, to come see her.

Mrs. Takata learned later on that Mrs. Shimura had been in a coma and dying of dysentery a few years earlier when a schoolmate of her daughter had told her about the Reiki Master, Dr. Chujiro Hiyashi. Mrs. Shimura's daughter sought Dr. Hiyashi's help and to everyone's amazement Mrs. Shimura came out of the coma and made a complete recovery. Thus, Mrs. Shimura took Mrs. Takata to Dr. Hiyashi's offices and two of his practitioners worked on her.

Mrs. Takata could feel warmth coming from their hands and looked under the table and at the ceiling to discover where the electrical cords were. Finding nothing, she surmised that they must have something up the sleeves of their kimonos and so she grabbed one of the sleeves. The startled man though she must be in need of a tissue and thoughtfully handed her one. Mrs. Takata questioned where the machine that made his hands so hot was hidden. When the man burst out laughing, Dr. Hayashi came over to see what the commotion was about because Reiki is usually done in silence or with quiet talking when necessary.

Dr. Hiyashi tried to explain the energy to Mrs. Takata; "All I know is that I have reached this great Universal Life Force and it comes through me to you to balance your system. These (he held up his hands) are the electrodes. It is similar to the radio waves that are sent out from the station and are picked up by the local receiving station which is the radio. We can't see them but we experience their effect."

After three weeks of daily treatments Mrs. Takata was so much better that she grew curious about learning how to do Reiki. In four months' time she was completely healed of all of her ailments and asked to be able to learn how to do the treatments. Dr. Hiyashi was reluctant to teach her because he felt that it should remain a secret within Japan. He felt that too much of the sacred Japanese culture had already been given to the Western World. Mrs. Takata sought the assistance of Dr. Maeda. He wrote to Dr. Hiyashi on her behalf and convinced Dr. Hiyashi to call a meeting of the directors of the association and get permission for Mrs. Takata to work with him.

Mrs. Takata spent months studying and eventually went out into the field to help others. She was unaware of the full reports of her progress that were being sent back to Dr. Hiyashi. As a result of these reports, Dr. Hiyashi allowed Mrs. Takata to become a Reiki Master.

Mrs. Takata's parents had returned to Hawaii after a year's stay in Japan, so she moved into the Hiyashi household to continue her studies. She stayed there for one year and did Reiki treatments every day.

In the summer of 1937, Mrs. Takata returned to Hawaii. A few weeks later, Dr. Hiyashi came to help her set up for classes on Reiki in Honolulu.

Dr. Hiyashi was an officer in the Japanese Naval Reserve and very concerned about an apparent threat of war. He knew that he would be called to active duty but as a devout Buddhist and the Reiki Grand Master, he could not kill people. He was only 62 years old and in perfect health when he decided to set a time for his own transition to occur. Dr. Hiyashi invited many people to come and at the agreed upon time he peacefully passed on. His body lay in state for seven days at the Reiki center and not one sign of deterioration was observed.

No one in his immediate family wanted to take on the daunting task of Reiki Grand Master, so Dr. Hiyashi had decreed Mrs. Takata to be his successor. She wanted to go back to Hawaii long enough to see her daughters grown and on their own and then she planned on going back to Japan and take over the Reiki clinic. In the meantime, World War II erupted and the two lost contact. Afterwards, Mrs. Takata returned to Japan to discover that the Reiki Center was the only building left standing in the midst of all the ruin. With that, it was decided that she would go back to Hawaii and spread Reiki to the rest of the world from her center there.

Through the intervention of war, this healing technique was brought from the East to the West and the number of practitioners grows daily.

In today's busy world it is not practical or often time possible to spend years in apprenticeship learning the ancient healing art of Reiki. Books of this nature are being produced by Reiki Masters in an effort to help with your learning process while keeping the sacredness alive. No longer are you required to go before a committee to be approved for learning Reiki. Your desire is qualification enough. No longer is Reiki a guarded topic. It is open and available to all who seek. But even so, it is my responsibility as a Reiki Master to remind you always of the sacred origination of this healing art and the importance of observing and respecting that tradition.

The Rediscovery of Reiki

In the mid 1800's Mikao Usui rediscovered and revived the art of Reiki healing. Many records were destroyed or lost during World War II and it may be that this is why there is no historical documentation of Usui.

It is said that he was a Buddhist monk and fluent in several languages, including Japanese, Chinese, English and Sanskrit. When he was questioned as to why man could not heal as Jesus and Buddha and other great religious leaders had said they could, he searched ancient Chinese writings for the answer. When he found none, he went to India to study their Holy writings.

Later, he returned to Japan where he discovered some Sanskrit formulas and symbols in ancient Buddhist sutras that appeared to hold the answers to his quest. He discovered some symbols but he did not know what to do with them or how to use them.

Usui decided to leave the monastery and go to the holy mountain of Kuriyama to fast and meditate in order to gain clarity on his questions. Hoping to gain contact with the level of consciousness needed to receive insight on the Sanskrit formula he had found, he fasted and meditated for 21 days. He kept track of his time there with the help of 21 stones which he placed in front of him and discarded at the rate of one per day.

During his twenty-one-day retreat, Usui read in the Sutras, sand and meditated but nothing happened until the morning of day twenty-one. Just before dawn he saw a distant light rushing toward him. He sat motionless as the light struck him in the forehead. He saw millions of little colored bubbles of light in all of the colors of the rainbow before a great white light appeared. Then large transparent bubbles appeared, each containing one of the symbols which he had discovered in the Sanskrit teachings. They paused long enough for him to commit to memory the instructions on how to use them; hence, the rediscovery of Reiki.

It took several hours for Dr. Usui to return to a normal state of consciousness. He was elated and felt a great strength and energy that would be abnormal after such a fast. He rushed down the mountain to share his news. In his haste he fell over a rock and noticed his toe was bleeding. He instinctively grabbed it in both of his hands and the pain and bleeding stopped within a few minutes. This was his first validation of the healing insights he had received.

Usui was hungry after his long fast and headed for a wayside inn where he ordered a large meal. Dr. Usui's beard growth and dirty array indicated to the inn keeper that he had been in meditative fast and he cautioned Usui to eat less to avoid adverse effects. But Usui ate all the food that was given him with no problems at all.

The food was served to Usui by the innkeeper's granddaughter, who was suffering from a toothache at the time. He asked permission to put his hands on her swollen face and when he did, the pain immediately ceased and the swelling went down. This was further validation of his newly discovered healing method.

After returning to the monastery, Usui decided the best use of his new healing skills would be in the slums of Kyoto where the poor beggars could be found. He felt that if he helped them feel better they could go out and earn a living instead of having to beg. After seven years Usui noticed that the same faces were showing up in the slums again. When he inquired of one of them as to why he had returned, the man answered that it was easier to beg than to try to work for a living.

Usui was deeply troubled to hear this and felt he had failed. It was then that he realized that he had forgotten one of the great principles of healing and that is the "attitude of gratitude" towards it. Thus in the days that followed he formulated these Reiki principles

Just for today do not worry.
Just for today do not anger.
Honor your parents, teachers and elders.
Earn you living honestly.
Show gratitude towards all living things.

Soon thereafter he left the slums and began traveling around Japan to teach Reiki. In order to attract to himself the right kinds of people, he would stand on a street corner holding a lighted torch in the middle of the day. Once he had gotten the attention of the people around him, he would invite them to attend a meeting at night if they really wanted to learn about the light. Many showed a desire and attended and in this way he was able to spread his teachings about this marvelous method of healing.

Mikao Usui is now buried in a Kyoto temple with the story of his life written on his gravestone. It is said that his grave is honored by the Emperor of Japan.

One of Mikao Usui's most dedicated students was Dr. Chujiro Hayashi. A Reserve Naval Officer, Hayashi was initiated into Reiki in the mid 1920's. He was given the title of Grand Master upon the transition of Mikao Usui. Dr. Hayashi moved forward with Reiki and opened a clinic in Tokyo. Because Dr. Hayashi was from a prominent family, he was able to attract the affluent and educated segment of Japanese society and even some of the nobility. This is where Mrs. Takata came in 1935 to eventually become the future grand master of Reiki and to bring it to the Western World.

Reiki and Raku-Kei

Raku-Kei is the art and science of spiritual self-improvement. It originated in Tibet and was practiced by the Tibetan Lamas. "Reiki" comes from Raku-Kei. Raku means the vertical flow of energy and Kei (or Chi in Chinese) is the horizontal energy. These two words, or calligraphs, were painted upon large wall hangings and were the focus for enlightenment for the Tibetan holy men. Participants sat on a four legged wooden stool that was placed in the center of an earthenware container. This container was oval in shape to represent the Akasa (etheric egg) and contained three inches of water. The stool was made wood with pure silver inlays going up the sides of each of the four legs. The inlays connected to a silver inlay cubicle on the seat.

One wall of the temple was a highly polished copper. Behind the aspirant was an angled wall that contained the Lama's prayer and the calligraphs of the Reiki symbols. These symbols were reflected by the copper wall and the initiate would reflect upon them while sitting on the stool. The purpose was to implant the symbols deep into the brain through concentration. By doing so, the consciousness and awareness of the individual was raised while the body and mind were purified. This very esoteric science that was passed down by word of mouth only eventually disappeared.

The Reiki calligraphs were used only for self-development and spiritual purification in the beginning. Many changes have taken place as a result of Usui's rediscovery of the system. Some revisions of them have been made in order to appeal to the Western Mind. To learn the true Reiki System, it takes many, many days of concentration and memorization along with exercises and postures.

The science of molecular biology can be applied to the concept of Reiki. The Reiki symbols have minute electrical energies that emanate from them. The second degree symbols have a powerful effect on the mind/body connection while the third degree symbol has the power of concentration in the formation of mental imagery.

In our study of quantum physics, we have learned that all matter is made up of energy and geometric designs, even when simply drawn on paper with a pen or a pencil, emit energies of various frequencies. Designs such as spirals, cones, crosses and abrupt right angles have molecular-electric influence on the neuro-muscular system of the body. The Reiki symbols also have this effect on physical structure. I was a healing facilitator long before I was attuned to Reiki. The most profound difference I noticed after being attuned to Reiki was the ability to do back to back healing sessions without the usual draining of energy that I experienced prior to receiving my attunement.

Channeling the Energy

Anyone can become a practitioner of Reiki. There is no barrier because of sex, race, creed, occupation or income level. You only need desire. Those who have received attunements from a qualified Reiki Master are able to proceed to help others with Reiki. It does not matter what level of Reiki a person is. Level I or Level II can be just as powerful as Mastership. (Level III). Level III practitioners should be those who want to teach and pass the information about Reiki on to others and there should be no stigma attached to those who just desire to do healing work instead of teaching it. The key is to have as many people using Reiki around the world as possible to help purify and balance it.

The healing energy of Reiki is transmitted through the hands and feet of the practitioner who has been attuned by a qualified Reiki Master. Reiki energy comes from the Source, Creator, Universe or whatever term you feel comfortable with. You, as the healing facilitator, should simply allow the energy to pass through you and into the recipient. In no way should you use your own energy, but simply allow this energy to freely flow through you. This is a very important factor because if you allow yourself to get in the way the Reiki energy becomes blocked and you will find yourself drained of energy. This experience is often referred to as an Empathic Drain. This is what I experienced prior to being attuned and I assure you it is exhausting! More than once I spent the following day in bed regaining my energy level.

It is important to remember that you never heal anyone. You are simply the healing facilitator. The recipient allows and accepts the balancing energy that promotes healing at whatever level it is needed. When the healing practitioner has a vested interest in the recipient he/she may be tempted to want to make it happen. The mind of the channel should remain null and void of the physiological or mental attitude and condition of the recipient. One of the hardest lessens to learn is that you cannot take away the free will of anyone and if it is for someone's highest band best good to remain ill or diseased then you must respect that fact. A person who receives Reiki is always helped, even if the outcome is not what the person or the channel wants or expects.

A normal Reiki session lasts about one hour. In severe or extreme cases the session could last longer. The recipient remains fully clothes and takes off his or her shoes and lies down. It is easiest to perform Reiki if you have a massage table available to you but a chair, couch or bed will do if need be. The Reiki channel sits or stands at the left side of the recipient and places his or her hands across the recipient's chest. It is not necessary to touch the recipient's body because you are channeling the energy and it will be absorbed either way. [If you plan on touching it is advisable to check your state laws on healing by touch.] If you do touch, use no pressure or manipulation.

The hands of the facilitator stay in one place until the area being treated stops drawing the energy. The energy flow will adjust itself automatically to the needs of the recipient. If the area requires a lot of energy, the flow will be felt very strongly by the facilitator.

The facilitator's fingers are held tightly together at all times. The facilitator starts at the head of the massage table and covers the appropriate positions on the head, including the eyes. At this time the practitioner would be sitting or standing at the head of the table behind the head of the recipient so that his or her fingertips would be pointing toward the recipient's feet when the hands are applied properly.

The facilitator (channel) moves his or her hands to the succeeding positions (shown in the treatment section) making sure to cover all points of the trunk of the body. Then he or she moves to the knees and then to the feet. Finally, the facilitator asks the recipient to roll over so that he or she can cover all points on the back of the torso.

There are those who say that jewelry or metal should not be worn during a Reiki treatment by either the facilitator or the recipient. Although I prefer to work without it, I was not taught that it could not be worn. If it were actually true that metal disrupted the flow of the Reiki energy then the healing table would be useless, as most tables have metal in them and you would have to be out of doors away from wires, etc. because houses have nails and wires and other types of metal material. I forgo jewelry strictly for personal preference. This is an area for you and the recipient to determine at the time of a session.

The recipient of a Reiki session may feel nothing at all, depending on how sensitive to subtle energy he or she may be. It has been my experience that the recipient primarily feels heat with an occasional reversal of feeling cold. The facilitator usually feels the energy as a warmth or heat that is often combined with a tingling sensation. This heat and tingling sensation dissipate as the energy is no longer being drawn. Although rare, in some instances the facilitator or the recipient may feel nothing at all and it is up to the facilitator to sense when it is time to move to another point. When the facilitator is unsure if energy is being drawn a good rule of thumb is to stay in a position for 5 minutes.

If the energy of the recipient is very out of balance the pull may be felt strongly by the facilitator. If the recipient is in balance the facilitator feels the pull much less. It takes a moment to determine if the energy is being drawn strongly or not. If after that amount of time, the facilitator feels or senses no energy is being drawn he or she should move to the next position.

The recipient should be advised to rise slowly from the healing table after a session has been completed. Many ties a lot of energy has been moved and he or she may feel very light headed for a few minutes as a result. Offering the recipient a glass of filtered water for grounding is recommended at this point.

This water will also serve to help the recipient's body eliminate any toxins that may have been released into the blood stream during the Reiki session. Encouragement to continue to drink filtered water throughout the next 24 hours is also advised.

Many times a Reiki session can result in sending the recipient into what is called a Healing Crisis. This is when the recipient seems to be getting worse instead of better. When pent up or imbalanced energy is finally addressed after many years, the body has to adjust to it and many times it is thrown out of kilter for a few days while this occurs. A healing crisis can take the form of worsened symptoms of the dis-ease that originated the desire for the Reiki session or diarrhea, or a "cold" or some other symptom that is really nothing more than the body's way of detoxifying itself. Although uncomfortable, a healing crisis is nothing to be alarmed about and should actually be considered a good sign.

People tend to literally hold issues in the tissues of their bodies and if something has been there for a long time it will most likely take a long time to release. When dis-ease has been around long enough to be considered chronic it will take time for the body to come back into harmony. Although you should always have hope and be positive, if a disease is considered terminal, Reiki may not be able to reverse it. This may be a case where that disease is the way the soul has chosen to leave the body and if that is so, the facilitator should step back and honor the soul's decision.

Remember, the sooner you apply Reiki to an illness or a dis-ease, the better. Accidents that have not yet had time to become cellular memory are easy to treat with Reiki.

You cannot make a mistake when performing a Reiki healing session. Reiki energy knows what to do. It has an intelligence of it own. Although you may be directing it into one receptive area it will go to the part of the body where it is needed. (I.E. You may be directing it into the feet and it will be helping the liver to heal itself)

Reiki energy comes from an intent to heal and the people come from and intent to be healed. On the physical level, when you touch or direct the energy, you heal. Try to keep one hand directing energy at all times while moving the other to a new position.

It is important that you keep your fingers together to help with the buildup and projection of energy. Do not let it eke through your fingers and flow randomly. Remember that you are the receiving tower of the energy and there is a massive continual exchange of energy between you and the recipient.

If you intend to do hands-on healing, it is important that you always ask for permission to do so. Remember that Reiki is just as effective without touch and if the recipient is not comfortable with touch he or she may block the flow of energy and diminish the effects of the Reiki session.

The left side of a person is considered the receptive side and the right side is considered the sending side. (This is why when you are in a circle you should always have your left hand up to receive energy and your right hand down to pass it on.) This is the reasoning behind standing at the left side of the recipient during a Reiki healing session, but in truth it makes minimal difference. Remember that you are working with energies so if you can blend with the chi of your surroundings all the better. If the table can be placed with the recipient's head facing north, wonderful. If not, don't worry – the session will still be powerful.

Don't be fooled into believing that nothing has happened after a Reiki session just because you or the recipient did not feel or notice anything. Something always happens. Always. There are many levels and layers to the body that are in need of balance and some are less likely to be experienced by the physical senses than others.

The body's suffering is a mask to hide what the mind is suffering. When you remove the cause, there shall be no effect. All dis-ease forms in the emotional body first. It is the body's way of getting your attention to let you know that something is amiss. Encourage recipients to listen to their own bodies and quit trying to put band aids on issues that need to be addressed. Covering them up will not cure them. By balancing the energy centers in the body, the emotions can be more readily handled and healed.

Congratulations! By now you have enough understanding about Reiki to receive Level I. The following positions should be practiced daily either on yourself or another person.

Head and Torso Hand Positions

Position 1.
Place hands over eyes.

Position 2.
Place hands over ears.

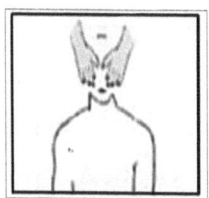

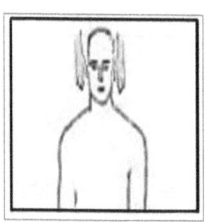

Position 3.
Place hands over back of head in V shape.

Position 4.
Place hands over throat

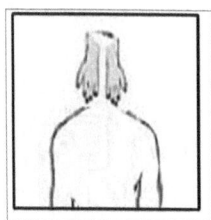

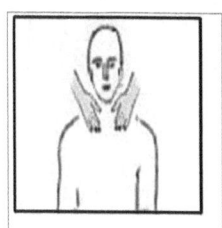

Position 5.
Place hands over collar bones.

Position 6.
Place hands over heart.

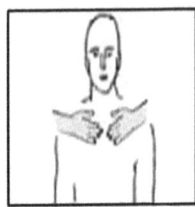

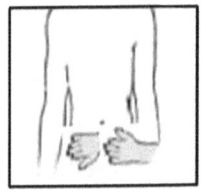

Position 7.
Place hands over Abdomen.

Position 8.
Place hands over stomach area.

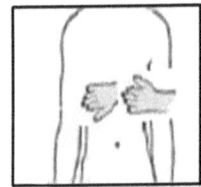

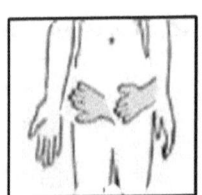

Position 9.
Place hands over groin area.

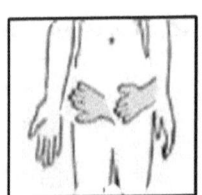

When Reiki Will Not Work

There will be times when Reiki does not seem to flow through the recipient and the recipient does not seem to get better. This can be due to a number of reasons- one being the fact that we expected a certain kind of reaction to occur and then the natural Law of Karmic Exchange took over and brought about something else.

Even though you may not see results this does not mean that something much deeper hasn't happened. Sometimes the energy simply allows certain repressed emotions or attitudes to surface later when they can be handled in private. Other times the recipient surprises himself or herself releases by saying something to someone that he or she has been holding in for a long time.

Often the recipient has no conscious idea as to what brought on the dis-ease. The subconscious mind holds the key to healing efficacy at all levels. When this is the case, counseling and guidance become necessary adjuncts to the Reiki treatment being performed. Encourage the recipient to listen to his or her own body and to just be aware of any new patterns of energy that may arise. Many times changes are very subtle and are missed in day to day living.

Do not be disappointed if your expectations are not fulfilled with certain clients. Remember that nothing is achieved with Reiki by force of will. The Ego has to take second place and make room for the Higher Self to open up and channel the Reiki energy.

You will find that many people cling to their illness. They actually own it. There are many reasons for this. Some feel it brings to them the attention they desire and don't get when they are well. Others use illness hide their fear of living up to certain expectations from the people around them. Whatever the reason, the Reiki can only help if the recipient allows it to. It is the recipient's responsibility to get well and it is your responsibility to offer them an avenue to take. You cannot will it or make it happen if the recipient truly does not want it.

Never push Reiki on a person. If the person is not eager to receive and learn it will only end up in disaster. The recipient has to be open to receive or your time and theirs is wasted.

The world is full of a variety of personalities, so it shouldn't come as a surprise when I tell you that you may run into some people who will actually ask for a Reiki session simply to prove to you, and themselves, that is does not work. And guess what. It won't. They have free will and final say of what happens with their body. If that is their mind set, they will block all efforts of channeling by lying on the table stiff, tense, skeptic and resist every flow of energy and pleasant sensation. They are also fighting any kind of harmony within the body.

Healing Plants and Animals with Reiki

Every living thing is made of energy, therefore every living thing can and will respond to Reiki energy. In fact, performing Reiki on an animal or a plant is made even easier since you do not have to overcome cultural or religious belief systems that might stand in the way of a smooth session.

When using Reiki on an animal you will notice that is gets very quiet and still. Many times it will come to be near you when you are giving treatments to others and especially when you are treating yourself. Reiki literally flows into animals exactly as it flows into people. When treating domestic animals, a good way to begin is to put your hands behind the ears at the point where dogs and cats like to be stroked. After this initial contact, then proceed to the afflicted areas of the animal's body or, if you are performing Reiki as a preventative measure, go to the chakra areas. (See Chakra Chart)

If you want to treat fish, you must place the aquarium between your hands and let the energy channel through for 15 to 20 minutes. This should be enough time to be quite effective.

When you start to channel Reiki into plants you will be impressed by the positive results you will get. Germany and Japan have been studying the effects of music and noise on plants for years. Music and noise are made up of energy. So, when you place Reiki energy into plants you will get noticeable results. Often the buds and blossoms are far more beautiful and healthy than non-Reiki plants.

To empower seeds that you are planting with Reiki

simply hold your hands a few inches above them or hold the seeds in your left hand and give them Reiki with your right hand. Cut flowers in a vase can also be made to last longer with the use of Reiki. Simply hold the Vase like you would when working with fish.

Potted plants are best treated through the root system. You do this by holding the pot between your hands near the bottom.

Trees can also be given Reiki. Trees take Reiki in through the trunk. Trees reciprocate in energy exchange. You have heard the saying; "Go hug a tree" had more validity than most people assume.

There are several planes of consciousness that all energy associates with. Even upon the higher planes there can be an exchange of energy. There is a plane of energy-consciousness where plants are able to express their gratitude for your channeling efforts. Be aware of this other type of plane-consciousness factor and open yourself to it. Once you have attained Reiki II you will know of symbols that, when activated, provide even a stronger and clearer channel of Reiki energy.

Horse Chakra Chart

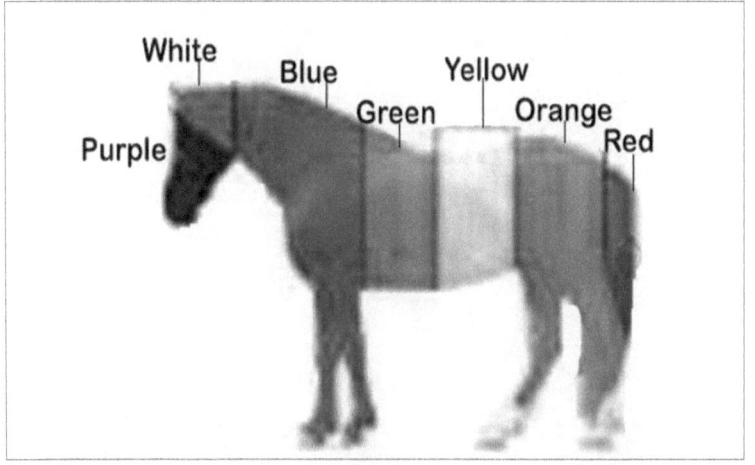

Dog Chakra Chart

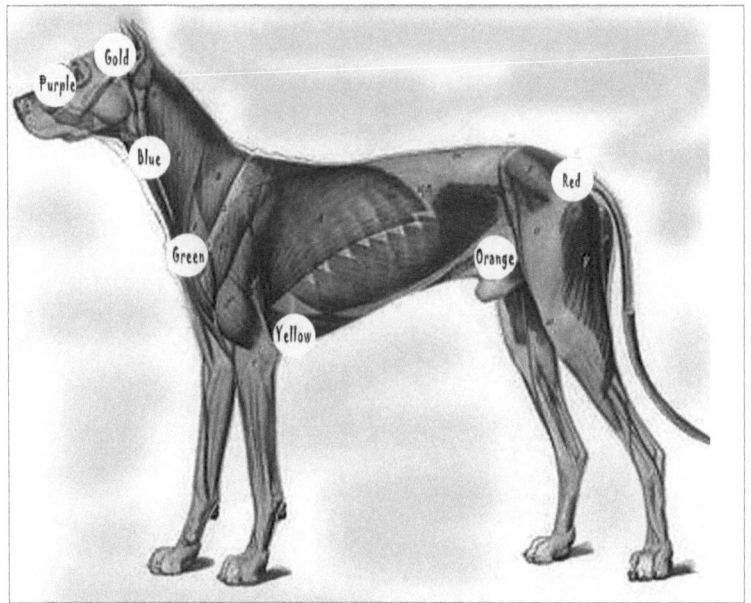

Kundalini

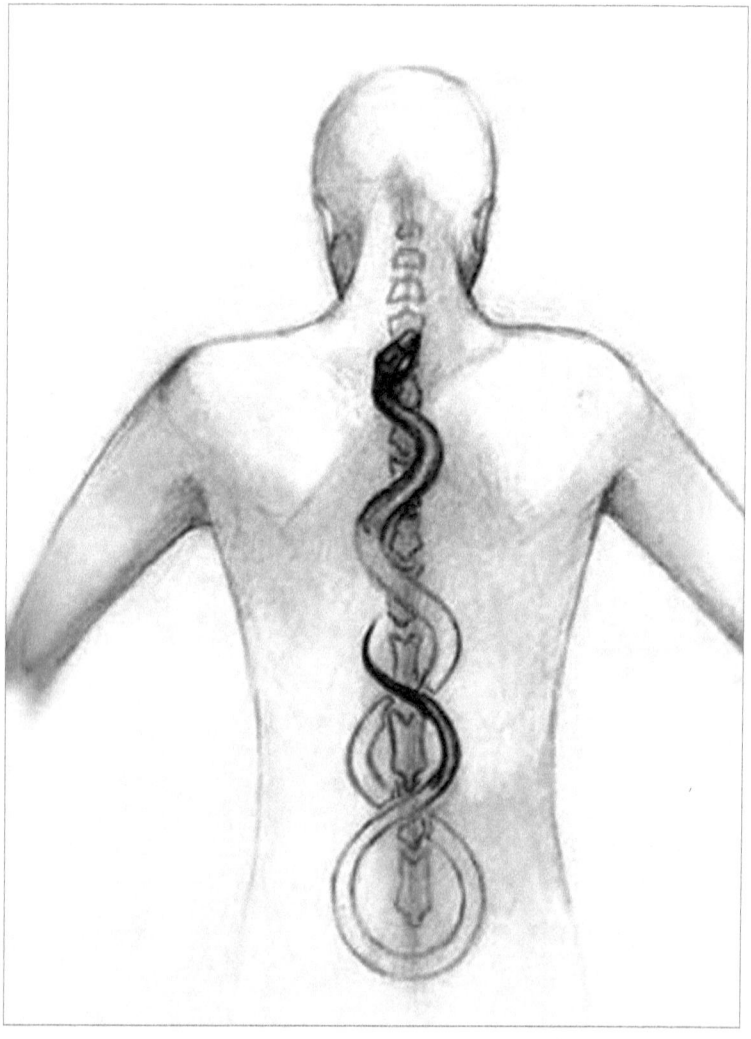

Human Chakra Chart

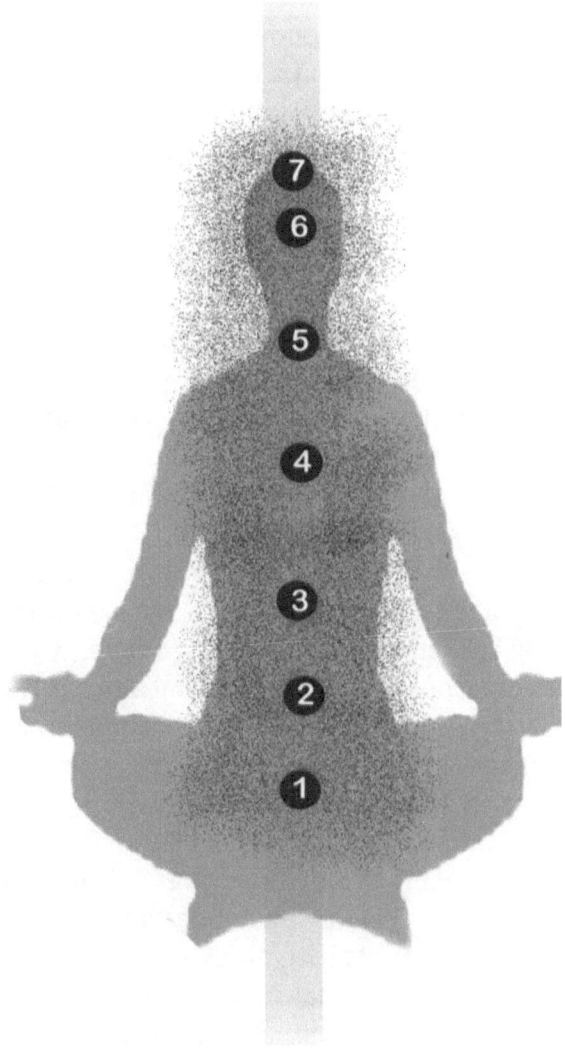

The Chakras

Although it is not imperative to know and understand the chakra system in a body in order to do a Reiki session it can prove beneficial.

Chakra is the Eastern term for what Westerner's call a Vortex or power opening. The work chakra is Sanskrit for "wheel". A human has hundreds of chakras on the subtle body, which is the counterpart for the physical one, but there are seven main ones that holistic healers and meditators focus on. Many with the gift of psychic sight are able to see the colored energy that radiates from each of these main chakras. Because we are all different, the colors are often viewed differently. For the purpose of this book I will give you the most common colors as well as the way I view them.

The lower three chakras represent the fundamental needs and emotions and vibrate at a lower frequency, thus being cruder in nature. The finer energy of the upper four corresponds to higher mental and spiritual aspirations. Excess or blocked energy from emotional causes in any chakra can result in dis-ease in the physical body. It is necessary that all chakras be balanced, as they are all equal in value. Too much emphasis on the upper four results in not being grounded, or being "out there" and too much attention on the lower ones leads to being very ego centered and not spiritually oriented.

The first vortex/chakra is the root chakra. It is perceived as the color red. This chakra is the survival center, the ability to draw abundance from the planet and is located at the base of the spine. It is the seat of physical vitality and it regulates those mechanisms which keep the physical body alive. It governs both survival and abundance issues. The Kundalini, or life force for survival, is located here and if not properly utilized, it results in fear or the constant fight or flight syndrome. This force lies dormant until the higher self can learn to properly release it and use it on both physical and spiritual levels. It is the endless source of power from Infinite Spirit of which we are an integral part on Oneness. This root charka's expression of energy is directly related to health. Holding on to old and negative patterns will cause an imbalance here. The glands and organs it represents are the Suprarenal glands and the kidneys, bladder and the spine.

The second vortex/chakra is perceived as orange and is located about two inches below the naval and is the center of sexual energy and the seat of creative power, feelings and emotions. First impressions and old emotional pictures are stored in this center. It is the proving ground for relationships. Creative vitality extends to all aspects of your life, not just to human reproduction and a block in this area leads to relationship problems as well as keeping you from realizing your good or your full potential in life. This center provides he pathway through which our spiritual co-creative powers take physical form. This is also the location of the Reiki point center, also known as the Hara or Tan Tien in martial arts such as Aikido. This chakra represents the gonads, reproductive organs and legs.

The third vortex/chakra is perceived as yellow located in just below the sternum, in the hollow between the two sides of the rib cage. It is the physical center of the body and is the place where physical energy is distributed. It is the seat of the will and some intuition which is why you often get a gut feeling about things. This chakra is commonly called the Solar Plexus. When there is a conflict between the upper and lower chakras this chakra will contract and there could be a literal tightening of the stomach. It is the center of unrefined emotions and the power urge; therefore, it is the power and wisdom center. The solar plexus represents the adrenals, the stomach, liver, gallbladder, pancreas and the digestive system.

The fourth vortex/chakra is in the heart area and is the color green. It is the connection between the upper and lower chakras, the intellect and emotions respectively. It is the seat of devotion and compassion trough which love, both conditional and unconditional, flows. It holds within it a connectedness to life. Ancient sayings state that God resides in this Chakra. Myth or fact, I like the thought. This chakra represents the thymus gland, and the organs it covers are the heart, the live, the lungs and the circulatory system.

The fifth vortex/chakra is in the throat area and is called the Throat Chakra. This chakra holds the master blueprint of physical wellness. It is the color blue or indigo. Since the vocal cords are located in the throat, this chakra is offered referred to as the communicative chakra. Many colds and sore throats are a result of not speaking your truth or not speaking up for yourself. Balancing of the throat chakra often brings forth thoughts and words that have been held back out of fear or dread. This chakra represents the thyroid gland and the throat, the upper lungs, arms and upper part of the digestive tract.

The sixth vortex/chakra is located in the forehead between the eyes and is perceived as purple or lavender. Psychics often refer to this chakra as the Third Eye because it is the area which they receive their visions. This gland represents the pituitary gland, the spine, the lower brain, the left eye, the nose and the ears as well as the hypothalamus and the autonomic nervous system.

The seventh vortex/chakra is located at the crown of the head. It is the one most connected to God and the Universal energies and represents the highest consciousness obtainable, enlightenment or I AM. It is often viewed as a golden ring around the head. This might explain the halos that are found in paintings of angles and saints. This chakra appears either gold or white. This chakra represents the pineal gland, the upper brain and the right eye.

Chakras, like the body, have a 24-hour clock rhythm. Although Reiki can be effect anytime, working with the flow of the chakra clock system will enhance and often intensify the effectiveness of the healing session.

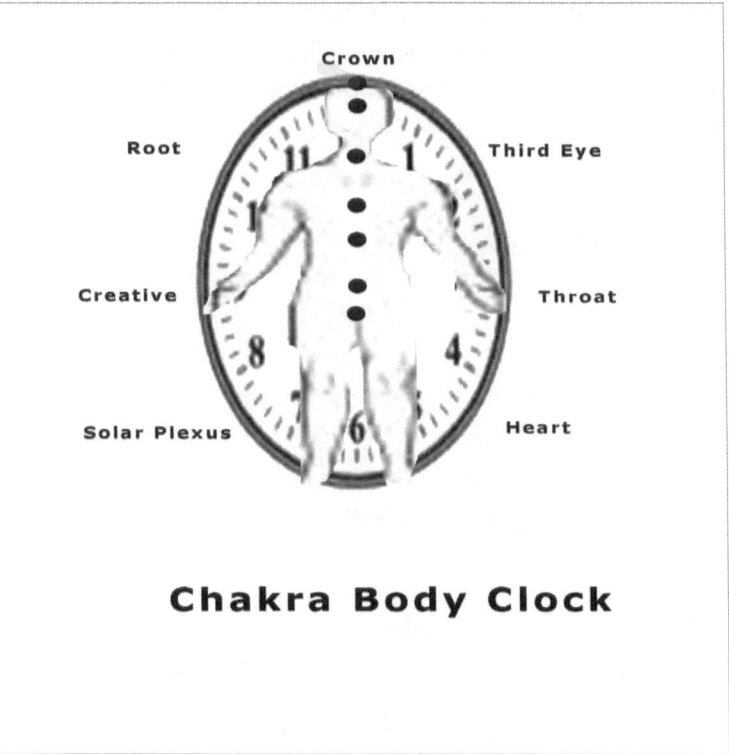

Chakra Body Clock

Reiki Level II

Second degree Reiki is for those who would like to add to their existing capabilities by sending long distance healing to others and boost the magnification of the healing energy that comes through them. The symbols, which are basically words in a language which is foreign to us, are very powerful and are not to be taken lightly. As soon as the symbols are drawn over the recipient's head, energy can be felt rushing through the giver to the receiver. Level II Reiki consists of a set of three Sanskrit/Japanese symbols with a vibration of the highest spiritual implication when utilized properly. Their names can be found in any Japanese-English dictionary. The last one, along with the Master symbol which is given in Level III Reiki, is pure Japanese kanji.

The symbols are as follows:

1. Cho Ku Rei (pronounced: cho koo ray)
Meaning:
• I am calling all the powers of the universe.
• Cho Ku Rei is Tibetan with a mixture of Indian Sanskrit. The circular shape represents a conch type shell symbolizing the calling to the heavens. It directs and focuses power.
• Cho – Curved sword, movement
• Ku – penetrating to make whole, whirlwind, spiral.
• Rei- universal soul, Spirit, mysterious power.
• Cho Ku Rei is the void. It cuts, penetrates and empowers. It is also used for transformation (dying) or leaving

this world.

2. Sei He Ki (pronounced: say hey key)

Meaning:

• Balance, karma, balance of the dynamics process of life
• Sei He Ki is Japanese.
• The symbol is used to align the body. It balances the upper four chakras mentally, spiritually and emotionally.
• Sei – the state of budding, getting there just before the opening (as in a flower's bloom)
• He – The base chakra of balance, foundation and origin of external form.
• Ki – energy, vital force, resonating to potential harmony, the hidden balance.

3. Hon Sha Ze Sho Nen (pronounced: Hone Shah Zay Show Nen)

Meaning:

• It is the bridge between two worlds. It is the ether tube connection for sending distant healing energy.
• Hon Sha Ze Sho Nen is Chinese.
• Hon – center, essence, origin, intrinsic nature.
• Sha – shimmering light.
• Ze – advancing, correct course, moving ahead.
• Sho – target, integrity, enlightened sage.
• Nen – stillness, the deepest part of.

When you use these symbols in healing, they should be visualized and drawn with hand movement at the same time. Every time you draw the Reiki symbols, strong elementary forces are activated.

In the original teachings of Reiki, once you were attuned to these frequencies you were engaged in a sacred vow not to reveal them to the uninitiated. Sense of honor prevailed and the symbols were only to be revealed to someone who has the proper training. But, in today's world that sacredness has been lost and there are many books, including this one, that have the symbols in bold print. Having the symbols in print helps with training in today's hectic and fast paced world but should in no way diminish the sacredness of them. The initiate should hold reverence to these sacred teachings and to those who come before him or her as is the ancient Reiki teaching.

Although this book aids with learning and understanding Reiki, it is still necessary to receive the attunements from a qualified Master Teacher of Reiki. During this attunement you will be taught the proper method to write the kanji in order to achieve them correctly.

The order of which you draw the symbols is as follows:
1. Cho Ku Rei
2. Sei He Ki
3. Hon Sha Ze Sho Nen

The Cho Ku Rei is what revs up the healing engine and gets things started. When I am going to perform a Reiki session on someone I draw the Cho Ku Rei in the room first, then on me and then on the person. Since it is tradition to keep the symbols sacred and hidden, I prepare the room and myself prior to having the recipient enter and then have the recipient close his or her eyes while I draw it over them. The Cho Ku Rei can be used by itself or with the other symbols. Remember that although you can use the Cho Ku Rei alone, the others must have it accompany them.

The Sei He Ki targets emotional issues. Since all dis-ease is rooted in the emotional body, I recommend always using the Sei He Ki.

The Hon Sha Ze Sho Nen is used when you are performing a remote healing. It is not necessary to use it if the recipient is in the room with you but it won't hurt anything if you do. Sending distant healing should be limited to 10 or 15 minutes.

Note: Although it is not necessary, many people like to use an object, like a teddy bear or a doll to help them visualize the absentee recipient.

Using Reiki II Symbols

Many tests and studies have shown that our bodies react to our thoughts. Applied kinesiology proves that as soon as we think of a negative thought, the biological organism reacts with weakness or reduced vitality. The same holds true for positive thoughts and actions. If you think a positive thought, you will bring forth strength and increased vitality. Reiki symbols increase the positive thought flow while providing a connecting light channel from sender to receiver. All dis-ease begins on the mental plane when our thoughts create little beings called elementals. These elemental thought forms whether positive or negative thrive and grow stronger both in consciousness and in physical manifestation.

You have access to all of these elementals and their power as well as to thought forms of all the prior Reiki practitioners who have come before you. Remember that thought is energy and energy can never be destroyed. Keeping this in mind, you have access to the wisdom of the ages!

A reminder that each Reiki symbol serves a specific purpose:
• The Cho Ku Rei serves to focus energy and to heal the physical.
• The Sei He Ki balances and aligns the upper four chakras and is for mental and emotional healing.
• The Hon Sha Ze Sho Nen is for distance healing.

To use and activate these symbols, draw it with

the flat of the hand, with fingers held tightly together, about one inch above the area that you want to treat or above the head of the recipient.

The pattern for a Reiki II healing is the same as a Level I. The only difference would be the drawing and activation of the Reiki Symbols. There is a basic formula of "start at the head and work your way down" but the actual pattern of energy placement may vary from person to person. I have supplied a commonly used pattern for "running the energy" [Creating a steady flow with not breaks. One hand is always focusing energy to the recipient) in this book but I encourage you to listen to your inner voice and the sensations you have flowing through you for the most effective Reiki session.

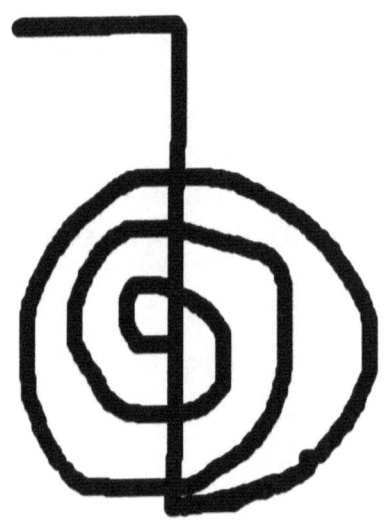

CHO KU REI

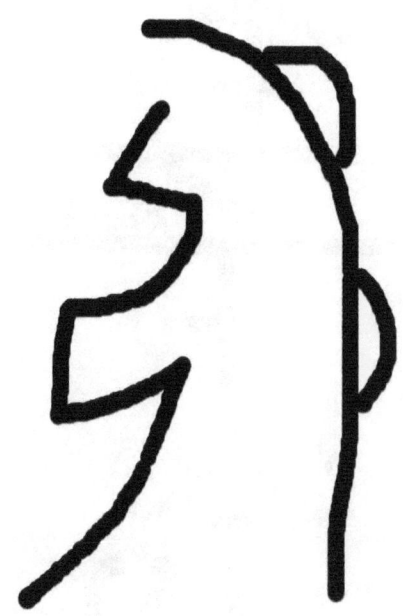

SEI HE KI

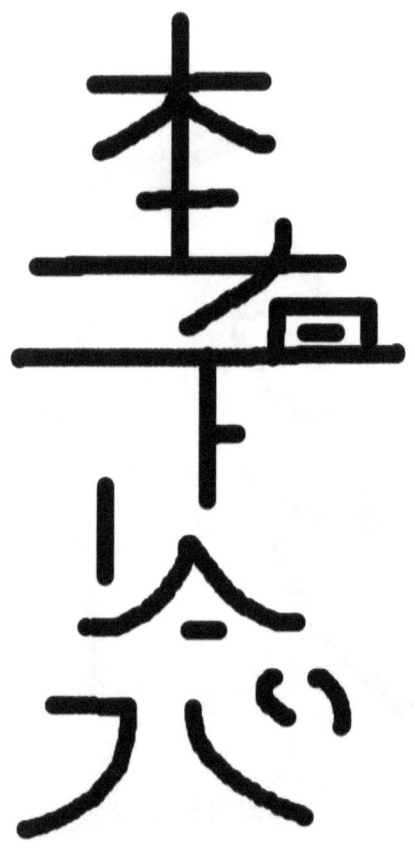

HON SHA ZE SHO NEN

Reiki Healing Pattern

The Hui-Yin Connection

There is a very close association between the chakra system and the endocrine glands. For thousands of years, initiates have been using the connection between the Hui-Yin point and the Governor Channel for spiritual transformation. By using the Hui Yin point properly, you can revert the Raku fire (Kundalini) up the spine and into the brain cells.

The first step in this process is known as Kidney Breathing. The majorities of the people I run into are literally breathing wrong and therefore are depriving their bodies of the true energy that is available to them. The proper way to breathe is to have the lower abdomen expand while in-haling and contract while exhaling. (Anyone who has played a wind instrument is aware of this method of breathing)

To learn how to do this method of breathing, place your hands directly over your kidneys on your lower back. Then take a nice slow, deep breath while you mentally direct the breath into the kidneys, visualizing it as a nice deep blue color. With every inhalation you should feel your hands moving away from you and with every exhalation your hands should be resting flat again. Eventually you will be able to keep your hands at your side while you perform this type of breathing.

To direct the Hui Yin, you must locate the acupuncture/ acupressure point that can be felt as a small sensitive hollow midway between the genitals and the anus. This area is the perineum and can be found pictured in any good anatomy book. Contract that area as long as possible (If you have done a Kegel exercise you will be fine doing this. If you need help with the contraction, place your finger on the area and press firmly.) Work up to a point where you can hold this contraction for as long as three minutes.

Once you have mastered the Hui Yin contraction and understand it, proceed with the following exercise:

1. Make the Hui Yin contraction tightly.

2. Press your tongue firmly against the roof of your mouth and maintain this pressure throughout the exercise.

3. Take a breath and expand your lower abdomen at the same time. Visualize your breath as a white mist going down through your body and collecting at the base of your spine. When you have completed the inhale, hold your breath and imagine it entering your spine at its base and rising up your spine like a hollow flute.

4. Still holding your breath, imagine the white mist entering your head from the top of your spine and swirling around clockwise inside your head and penetrating your brain. Visualize the white mist turning blue inside your head and turn it into a clear violet color. Hold this image and your breath for about two minutes (if possible) and then resume normal breathing.

5. Repeat the entire process two more times.

Learning to hold your breath and the contraction as long as possible is the essence of this energy accumulation and it gives a tremendous self-energy charge that sometimes manifests as alight-headedness. This type of manifestation will pass with time, practice and dedication.

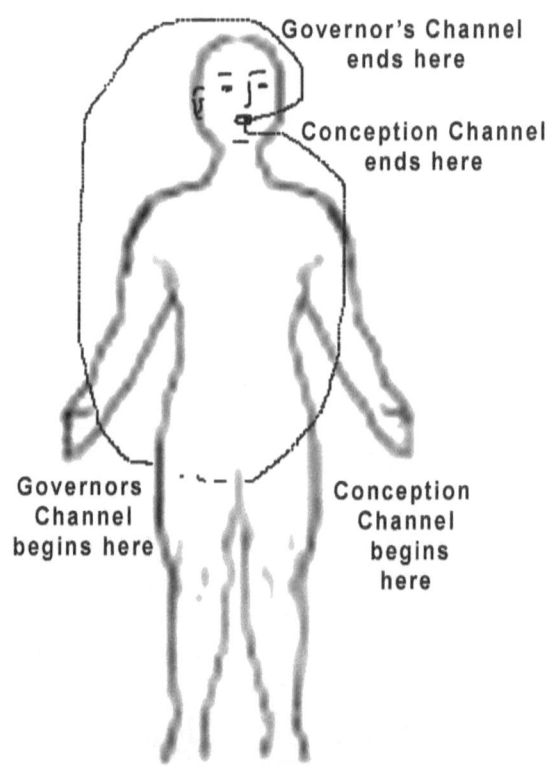

The Hui Yin Connection

After Your Attunements

Each attunement that you go through changes your vibratory rate to a higher level. As is shown by the science of quantum physics, everything on earth is just matter in motion, or energy. Atoms in molecules are constantly in motions so that even things which appear to be solid to us are in a state of constant slow motion. As a vibratory rate is raised, it becomes less dense. My favorite example is water, air and ice. Ice is a very slow vibration but when you speed it up a little it will melt and take the form of water. Speed the water vibration up and it will turn to steam and then disappear into the air.

In the same way, you raise your vibrations by undergoing each Reiki attunement. When you do this, you cast off the old and negative energies that you have been holding onto and you start a 21-day cleansing process.

It takes three days for the energy to go through each of the seven chakras, starting at the root chakra and working up to the crown. During this time, you may experience very subtle or extremely strong changes in your life. If you have issues in certain areas, as the energy goes through the corresponding chakra it will bring these issues up for you to deal with. Most of us who are into healing are very glad to have those old stored up emotions and memories released.

For most people these changes are easily handled. A few are thrown into a healing crisis, but that too subsides after the three days. Always remember that emotions are energy also. Some of the changes you might observe would be things like having strange dreams that you remember, having heightened sense of intuition or that gut feeling, about what is going on with yourself or other people, or find that a favorite food or habit suddenly loses its importance in your life.

Many Reiki practitioners find that they cannot be around very negative people anymore. Their circle of friends generally makes a shift. Excessive alcohol is one thing that will greatly lower a person's vibration and many practitioners note that they can no longer drink alcohol or stand to be around those who do. Life becomes easier if you seek out others who are of like mind. It just makes sense.

Some reactions may seem to be difficult or unpleasant at first but remember that they are temporary. If you maintain not attachments to the results, you will be better able to just say "yes" to each experience and go on about your business.

Changes can often times be very subtle and it may take a friend or family member to point it out to you. I suggest you keep a daily journal so that you can reflect back on your changes later on and/or share with a recipient who may be experiencing a healing crisis.

It is helpful to Reiki yourself either before you go to sleep at night or when you first wake up. By doing so, it will help you to move out any undesirable energy in your body plus give you more practice on the hand positions. It will also accelerate growth and further refine your energy which will bring more abundance into your life.

The Attunements

As with Level I and Level II of Reiki, you should wait a minimum of twenty-one days before you receive your attunement. Historically, it took years before an individual was allowed to become a Reiki Master, not days.

The following is the attunement method for Levels I, II & III:

The initiate should be sitting in a chair, eyes closed, hands in prayer position. The Master greets the initiate from the front with a traditional bow and then moves to the back of him or her. (Always go counter-clockwise around a person)

1.   Have your predominant hand over the initiate's head and with your other hand draw the Cho Ku Rei in the air while visualizing it and forming the words with your lips (or softly whispering them). Then, with your predominant hand, draw the Dai Koop Mayo over the crown Chakra with the tail of the symbol going down the spine.

2.   Next put both hands over the crown chakra while visualizing and saying the Cho Ku Rei, Hey Se He Ki and Hon Sha Zen Show Nan.

For the rest of the attunement, both hands are to be in the following positions while visualizing and saying Dai Koop Mayo, Cho Ku Rei, Se He Ki and Hon Sha Zen Show Nan (respectively):

a. Hands on shoulders

b. Hands on inner shoulder with thumbs touching the spine

c. On right side of initiate: right hand on forehead and left hand at the base of his/her skull

d. On right side of initiate: hold initiate's hands together with the left hand and have your right hand fingers touching where the initiate's fingers touch each other (still in prayer position)

e. Go to the front of the initiate and bring his or her fingers up to touch his or her brow chakra (forehead). While breathing in, draw the Cho Ku Rei with your tongue and say/visualize the symbol in your mind. Breathe out in short quick breaths and focus the breaths at the crown, brow, throat and heart chakras. Note: Breath at the throat and heart chakra is done below the initiate's hands so that the initiate's fingers are still touching his/her brow chakra.

f. Place both of the initiate's hands on his/her lap and gently let him/her know the process if finished.

Level II & Level III

The following is to be added for Level III attunements:

Just before step C above, go to the front of the initiate and place one of the initiate's hands on his/her lap while holding the other one and drawing the Cho Ku Rie, Se He Kei and Hon Sha Ze Sho Nen over the palm of the initiate's hand. Note: After drawing each symbol gently tap it into the palm before drawing the next. Place the first palm down on the initiate's lap and gently lift the other hand and repeat. When you have completed this, take both of the initiate's hands and gently return them to the prayer position and proceed to step C above.

The following is to be added for Level III only:

When following the instructions for Level II include the Dai Koo Myo when drawing the symbols over the initiate's hands.

Reiki III is also the Mastership Level. This level is only necessary if you wish to teach Reiki to others and pass on the attunement. Otherwise, it is perfectly fine to remain a Level II practitioner. The Mastership symbol that is imbued in you will not make you a stronger or clearer channel of Reiki energy than a Level II practitioner.

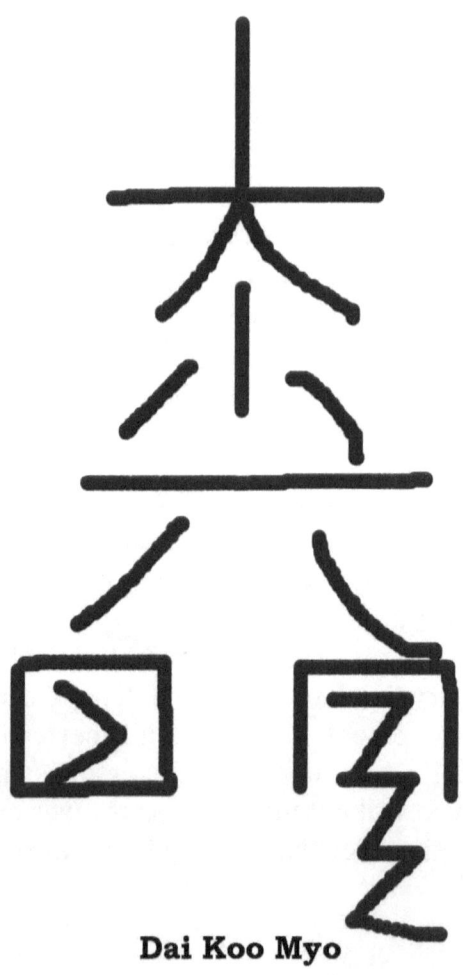

Dai Koo Myo

Dai Koo Myo   (Master Symbol)

The Tibetan way of the Fire Serpent incorporates the rising of the Serpent (Kundalini) energies up the spine, culminating in the Crown. Once you have raised your vibration you should strive to keep it there by being aware of your diet and activities. It may be that you can no longer eat certain food or drink certain beverages or be in certain places without having a pretty severe reaction to the low density of vibrations found there. Just be aware and listen to what your body it trying to tell you.

The Sui Ching water ritual has been an integral part of the Fire Serpent initiation in Tibet for thousands of years and is taught in Tibetan monasteries. I point out again that in the beginning of Reiki; it was used for spiritual self-improvement and not taught as a healing modality. The Sui Ching method can be used to energize your water or food prior to ingesting it.

Water binds itself to magnetic energy and mediates all chemical and physical processes inside and outside the body's cells. Just as water takes on surrounding smells, it can be loaded with magnetic energy. When water is charged with this magnetic energy from human organisms it takes on a taste very different from normal water. When you drink magnetized water, sick or sensitive people sometimes perceive a characteristic smell or taste of steel or sulfur.

Water contains spirit frequencies of 106 electron count. The human body, being 75% water, also contains this spiritual frequency. Contaminated water contains no spiritual frequency. It is imperative that contaminated water NOT be used during an attunement. When attuning to Reiki, water treated and magnetized by the Sui Ching method should be supplied by the Reiki Master.

How to treat Water with the Sui Ching Method

First obtain a bottle of purified or filtered water that has not been opened. (Tap water is not suitable for this exercise) Turn the bottle over and put it between your knees to hold it. Then place your hands, one above the other, about 4 inches above the container and rotate them counterclockwise in a circular motion while pressing your tongue against the roof of your mouth. (You are forming a vortex or gravitational field around the water). Rotate your hands smoothly for about 4-5 minutes. This will result in a partial vacuum in the center of the water which draws atoms toward the vortex. (Inertia in the center of the water draws energy into the field you have created) This is the type of water you must use in attunements for a high self-connection with your students.

Once the water has been activated, the student should drink at least part of it during the initiation process and the rest within a short period of time after the attunement. This activated water may be improved by adding fresh lemon juice, which cuts the mucus in the system and helps in absorbing the cosmic rays.

Now that you have learned about Reiki and have become attuned to it by a qualified Reiki Master. Please don't waste your knowledge. Go out and use it to help yourself and your loved ones.

About the Author

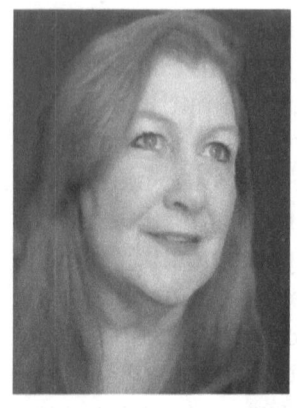

Lena Sheehan was born and raised in Upstate New York. Born with the ability to see and connect with the other side and gifted with all of her psychic abilities intact, she dediated over 24 years to Spiritual and Holistic care and management of body, mind and spirit. Feeling strongly that a balanced connection between an individual's body, mind and spirit is needed in order to achieve an optimum life experience, Lena has developed distance learning courses as well as private and group programs that work with all three.

An internationally known Visionary, Psychic Medium, and Spiritist, she holds a diploma in Traditional Naturopathy, is a Nutrition Specialist, a Hypnotherapist, the Founder of Haymanootha Healing (also referred to as The Sheehan Technique of Healing), a Reiki Master, a Karuna Ki Master, a Reflexologist and an Ordained Evangelistic Minister,(the Lively Stones Fellowship an evangelistic ministry, founded by Dr. Willard Fuller and an Interfaith Minister Director for the Universal Brotherhood Movement, Inc. (founded by Rick and Jeni Prigmore). Rev. Sheehan has authored multiple books and learning courses. She has been an ongoing guest of various radio stations in the Hudson Valley and Southern Tier, New York throughout the years; doing live call-in show. Her lectures, classes and workshops are primarily based on the information in her books and have been received by or offered through many private individuals as well as such places as:

*Holistic Haven #1, Johnson City, NY
*Holistic Haven #2, Scranton, PA
*Broome Community College, Binghamton, NY
*Broome County Hospice, Binghamton, NY
*Poughkeepsie Chamber of Commerce,   Poughkeep
   sie, NY
*New Paltz Chamber of Commerce, New Paltz,NY
*Health, Relaxation and You, Poughkeepsie, NY
*Center for Personal Development, Wappingers
   Falls, NY
*Seeds of Light Learning Center, Fishkill, NY
*Estrella Mountain Community College,Avondale, AZ
*The Arizona Enlightenment Center,Goodyear, AZ
*Mystic Moon Bookstore, Scottsdale, AZ
AZ Holistics, Tempe, AZ

For more information on Lena Sheehan go to:
 http://www.lenainc.com

or

For more information on books authored
by Lena Sheehan go to:
http://www.sheehan-author.info